Your Skin:

A step-by-step guide to creating the ideal skincare routine

By

Dr. Rebecca Mistry

TABLE OF CONTENTS

INTRODUCTION

The present generation is more concerned with their health, especially maintaining a regular skincare routine. A rigorous skincare regimen will keep your face looking bright and fresh, regardless of pollution or other environmental factors. It eliminates excess oil and debris from your pores regularly, which prevents the formation of acne, reduces sunspots, and makes your skin seem bright and plump.

Skincare is an important approach for maintaining the health of the skin on your face and body. A regular skincare regimen will help you maintain a healthy and youthful appearance. Several proteins must be integrated into your everyday skincare regimen, from washing your face to applying moisturizer. Understanding this can help you keep your skin looking young.

This book will teach you easy tactics and recommendations for creating your daily skin regimen. Sit back, relax, and wait for this game-changing tactic.

CHAPTER 1
GETTING TO KNOW YOUR SKIN

Understanding the four different types of skin: normal, dry, oily, and mixed.

Normal, dry, oily, and mixed skin are the four basic types of healthy skin. Hereditary factors influence skin type. Our skin's state, on the other hand, can vary substantially depending on the many internal and external stimuli to which it is exposed.

PERFECT SKIN

What Exactly Is Normal Skin?

The term "normal" is frequently used to describe well-balanced skin. Eudermic skin is the technical term for well-balanced skin. The T-zone (forehead, chin, and nose) is a little greasy, but overall sebum and moisture levels are balanced, and the skin is neither very oily nor overly dry.

How to Recognize Normal Skin.

Normal skin has the following characteristics:

- Fine pores

- Good blood circulation
- A velvety, silky, and smooth texture
- A fresh, pink tone uniform transparency
- No blemishes
- And is not prone to sensitivity.

A person with normal skin may experience dryness as they age.

SKIN IS DRY

What Exactly Is Dry Skin?

The term "dry skin" refers to skin that produces less sebum than normal skin. Dry skin lacks the lipids required to retain moisture and build a protective screen against environmental stimuli due to a lack of sebum. As a result, the barrier function is impaired. Dry skin comes in a variety of degrees of severity and unique morphologies that are not always obvious.

Women have far more dry skin than men, and all skin becomes drier as it ages. Dry skin problems are a common complaint, accounting for 40% of dermatologist appointments.

The Causes of Dry Skin

Skin moisture is determined by the availability of water in the deeper skin layers as well as sweat.

Skin regularly loses water through:

- **Perspiration:** which is an active water loss from the glands triggered by heat, stress, and exercise.

- **Trans-Epidermal Water Loss (TEWL):** a natural, passive mechanism by which skin diffuses around half a liter of water every day from deeper skin layers.

Dry skin is caused by a shortage of:

- Natural Moisturizing Factors (NMFs): which are mostly urea, amino acids, and lactic acid.
- Ceramides, fatty acids, and cholesterol are epidermal lipids that are required for a good skin barrier function.

As a result, the skin's barrier function may deteriorate.

How to Identify Different Levels of Dry Skin

Dry skin ranges from somewhat drier than normal skin to very dry skin and severely dry skin. In general, the discrepancies can be recognized by:

Skin Dehydration

Mildly dry skin can feel tight, fragile, and scratchy, as well as seem dull. The suppleness of the skin is likewise reduced.

Extremely Dry Skin

If the skin is not treated for dryness, it may develop:

- Mild scaling or flakiness in spots
- Rough and blotchy look (sometimes seems prematurely aged)
- Tightness
- Itchiness is a possibility.

It is also more susceptible to irritation, redness, and infection risk. Learn more about dry skin.

Very Dry Skin

Certain body parts, notably the hands, feet, elbows, and knees, are prone to:

- The roughness
- Chapping with a proclivity to create rhagades (cracks)
- Calloused skin
- Itching regularly

Extremely dry skin is most typically noticed in the hands of the elderly or those who are extremely dehydrated. Learn more about rough and cracked skin on the body.

SKIN THAT IS OILY

What Exactly Is Oily Skin?

The term 'oily' refers to a skin type with excessive sebum production. Seborrhea is the medical word for excessive production.

The Causes Of Oily Skin

Several causes contribute to sebum overproduction:

• Genetics

• Hormonal fluctuations and imbalances

• Medication

• Stress

• Comedogenic cosmetics (inflammatory cosmetics)

What are the different forms of oily skin?

Oily skin is identified by the following characteristics:

• Enlarged, clearly visible pores

• A gleaming sheen

• Thicker, paler skin: blood vessels may be obscured.

Oily skin is prone to comedones (blackheads and whiteheads) and acne of various types.

Mild acne causes a large number of comedones to appear on the face, as well as the neck, shoulders, back, and chest.

Papules (little bumps with no evident white or black head) and pustules (medium-sized lumps with a prominent white or yellow dot at the center) appear in moderate and severe instances, and the skin becomes red and inflamed.

SKIN COMBINATION

What Exactly Is Mixed Skin?

The skin types in mixed skin differ in the T-zone and the cheeks. The so-called T-zone can range in size from very tiny to extremely large.

Combination skin is identified by the following characteristics:

• Excessive oil in the T-zone (forehead, chin, and nose)

• Enlarged pores in this location, most likely due to contaminants

• Dry to normal cheeks

The Origins Of Mixed Skin

The oilier areas of mixed skin are caused by an excess of sebum. The drier areas of mixed skin are caused by a lack of sebum and a corresponding lipid deficit.

SKIN TYPE AND CONDITION EVALUATION

Skin condition, unlike skin type, may change substantially over your life. Climate and pollution, medication, stress, hereditary factors that influence the levels of sebum, sweat, and natural moisturizing factors that your skin produces, as well as the products that you use and the skincare choices that you make, are among the many internal and external factors that determine its condition.

Skincare products should be chosen to match skin type and condition. Dermatologists and other skincare specialists assess a person's skin type by taking into account the following factors:

AGE-RELATED SIGNS

Our skin type might change during our lives. Those with oily skin in their adolescence may notice their skin growing drier after puberty, whereas those with typical skin may see their skin becoming drier as they age.

Skin loses volume and density as it ages, fine lines and wrinkles emerge, and pigmentation changes might occur. Understanding and monitoring these aging markers allows us to assess the state of our skin.

SKIN TONE

Skin color and ethnicity have an impact on how our skin reacts to environmental factors such as the sun, pigmentation disorders, irritation, and inflammation. The density of the epidermis and the dispersion of melanin define basic skin color.

The appearance of skin redness Is also a valuable indicator of skin condition; it reflects how well our circulation is working and may aid in the identification of disorders such as couperose and rosacea.

SENSITIVITY OF THE SKIN

Sensitive skin is skin that is readily irritated by variables that are normally accepted by well-balanced skin, such as skin care products or extreme hot and cold temperatures. Sensitive skin is a persistent condition for some people, while for others, it is triggered by internal and environmental circumstances. It happens when the skin's natural barrier function is impaired, resulting in water loss and irritant penetration. Sensitive skin is more readily irritated and reactive than regular skin. Identifying and analyzing signs such as redness, a rash,

stinging, itching, and burning aid in the diagnosis of skin conditions. Symptoms are aggravated by variables that the face skin is most exposed to, such as the sun and certain substances in cosmetics and cleansers.

PRODUCTION OF SEBUM AND SWEAT

The amount of sebum generated by the skin's sebaceous glands regulates the efficiency of the skin's barrier function and, as a result, the skin's state. Overproduction of sebum can result in oily, acne-prone skin, whereas inadequate sebum production results in dry skin.

The glands of perspiration Sweating is produced by the skin to assist the body in maintaining its optimal temperature. Sweating excessively or seldom might have an impact on skin condition.

NMFs (NATURAL MOISTURIZING FACTORS)

NMFs, such as amino acids, are naturally formed in healthy skin and serve to bind water into the skin, retain its elasticity and suppleness, and keep it from getting dehydrated. When the skin's protective barrier is compromised, it is frequently unable to maintain these critical NMFs, causing skin moisture to diminish and condition to deteriorate.

CHAPTER 2

BASICS OF SKINCARE

Though everyone has different skin — and hence different skin issues, worries, goals, and so on — certain basic skin-routine guidelines apply to everyone. These are known as the fundamentals, and we visited several doctors to check what they are and provide skin-care recommendations that apply to all of us, novices and experts alike. If you're unsure how to put together a skin-care regimen (no judgment), or if you want to brush up on the fundamentals, this is your expert-backed beginner's guide to skincare.

The most Important skin-care tip is to keep things simple. Begin with the fundamentals and work your way up.

These necessities should always contain the three processes listed below, accomplished in the order listed:

Step1: Cleanse

The basic rule of thumb is to wash your face twice every day, once in the morning and once in the evening. Cleansing in the morning might assist in eliminating any perspiration or oil that may have accumulated on your pillow and hair throughout your restful sleep.

The twice-daily guideline has one common exception: dry skin. It's fine to take plain water in the morning if you're prone to dehydration.

Evening skin cleansing, on the other hand, should never be compromised or skipped. At the end of the day, washing is required to remove not only the skin-care products and cosmetics applied in the morning, but also excess oil, perspiration, dead skin cells, pollutants, and other debris that accumulate on the skin during the day.

Experts advise novices to choose a gentle, hydrating cleanser when selecting a face cleanser. A hydrating cleanser is suitable for all skin types. Look for one that is fragrance-free, has few chemicals (to decrease irritation), and contains ceramides and glycerin to repair and maintain the skin barrier.

Step 2: Moisten

After that, use a moisturizer or moisturizing lotion. "I usually recommend an oil-free, fragrance-free moisturizer," since it is well accepted by [all] skin types, from acne-prone to sensitive.

Aside from these characteristics, you may use this phase to concurrently treat certain skin issues by locating a moisturizer designed with extra constituents that target specific needs. The list of skin-care ingredients is extensive and ever-changing; thus, for the sake of this book, here are some of the most significant ones to be aware of as they apply to moisturizer:

• Hyaluronic acid: Rehydrates and plumps the skin.

• Ceramides: Important for skin barrier strength and general health (especially in persons with dry skin and eczema).

• Vitamin C: Promotes skin whitening and antioxidant protection.

If you have oily or acne-prone skin, don't believe you can (or should) forego using a moisturizer regularly. "Over-washing without the proper use of a moisturizer will produce an over-production of oil on your skin." Regardless of how oily or acne-prone your skin seems, it will dry up without replenishment, and dry skin is irritated skin.

People with oily skin, on the other hand, should look for noncomedogenic moisturizers. The term noncomedogenic on a product label means that the ingredients will not clog pores and cause further outbreaks.

Step 3: Safeguard

Your first line of defense and prevention against skin cancer is sunscreen. Sun protection is the most important thing you can do for your skin.

Choose an SPF 30 or higher sunscreen and apply it every day (even when it's cloudy), always as the last step in your skin-care regimen. EltaMD UV Active Broad-Spectrum Sunscreen 50+, Supergoop Glowscreen SPF 40, and Coppertone Pure & Simple Sunscreen Lotion for Face SPF 50, which is designed particularly for sensitive skin, are all fantastic choices.

When deciding on a sunscreen, there are two options: chemical or mineral-based (in some cases, both are merged into one composition). Mineral sunscreens act as a barrier, preventing the sun's rays from reaching the skin, thanks to ingredients such as zinc oxide or titanium dioxide. Chemical sunscreens, on the other hand, protect the skin from UV radiation by absorbing it and rely on substances like octocrylene or avobenzone to do so.

Add More Phases If Needed (Or Desired).

Once you've mastered the fundamental pattern, you may start adding new levels as needed. Exfoliation is a great place to start, adding it in as an extra step once or twice per week using alpha hydroxy acids (AHAs) or beta hydroxy acids (BHAs), which work in different ways to slough off undesirable deposits on the skin's surface.

There are two types of exfoliation treatments to choose from, just like there are two types of sunscreen. AHAs and BHAs are chemical exfoliants that are great for promoting cell turnover, increasing collagen production, and reducing dullness. Physical exfoliation, on the other hand, is exactly what it sounds like removing dead skin cells, excess oil, and buildup with a face scrub. Physical exfoliants should be avoided by

people with sensitive skin since they can irritate the skin and perhaps cause blood vessel damage.

Serums and masks are two additional add-on stages that you may rotate in and out of your program as required. Facial serums are high-potency, lightweight topicals that include a greater concentration of active ingredients, such as vitamin C and hyaluronic acid, to address more specific skin concerns. They should be used beneath your moisturizer; a common rule of thumb is to apply thinner items beneath heavier ones, such as moisturizers and oils.

You may also use a facial mask on occasion, but I recommend doing so no more than once or twice each week. Face masks should be used regularly, and should be applied to clean, dry skin. Look for a face mask that is designed to cure any skin issues you are experiencing that day; popular examples are hydrating, clarifying, relaxing, and brightening masks.

KEEP THESE IMPORTANT HINTS IN MIND.

Less Is More In This Case.

As your skin-care routine evolves and expands, maybe the most important thing to remember while slathering on cosmetics is that less is frequently more. Paring down your regimen and sticking to essential, necessary active ingredients will serve you far better than doing too much. Stick to products with few ingredients that are fragrance-free, and test new items one at a time to see how your skin reacts.

Be Patient.

If a new skin-care routine doesn't seem to be "working" right away, remember that patience is required when it comes to skincare (and be wary of any product that claims speedy results). Experiment sparingly. Allow your skin at least two to three months to adjust to a new product

or active ingredient before switching. The caveat here, of course, is that if a skin-care product causes irritation or an allergic response, discontinue usage immediately.

The Importance Of Consistency

Maintain consistency, which ties back to the patience factor. Consistency — going through the same skin-care regimen steps every day, morning and night — is critical to achieving and maintaining genuine results. Bottom line: Have faith in the process (and in yourself), and stick to whatever plans you make for yourself.

CHAPTER 3
THE VALUE OF A SKINCARE ROUTINE

6 REASONS WHY A SKINCARE ROUTINE IS ESSENTIAL

Our skin is a great organ, but it does require some assistance from time to time, which is where a skincare regimen comes in – and we're all about keeping it simple.

Here are the main advantages of having a healthy skincare regimen and how to get started.

1. Our Skin Appreciates Consistency.

The key word in skincare is consistency. Our skin desires it, and sticking to a skincare program for a month or longer can provide better results. This is because our skin cells renew every 28 days or so.

The good news Is that skincare does not have to be complicated. The goal is to wash, protect, and hydrate the skin. A cleanser, serum, and moisturizer are all you need for your face every day, plus an exfoliation once or twice a week. Your body needs to be pampered, so choose a body wash, scrub, and lotion that you love, and extra points if they're all-natural!

2. Our Skin Requires Help

Did you know that the skin is the body's largest organ? It is extremely defensive and spends the majority of its timekeeping irritants out, such as pollution and smoke fumes. While it performs an excellent job of safeguarding us, it cannot accomplish everything. That is why

establishing a skincare regimen is essential, as is using natural skincare to avoid adding to your body's harmful load.

Each skincare product is designed to perform a certain purpose, all to improve the health of your skin. For example, our skin does not clean itself, thus cleansers and body washes are necessary. They work to unclog our pores and remove impurities like oil, dirt, and grime from our skin. Moisturizers strengthen our skin's barrier, which not only protects against free radicals that cause premature aging but also lowers inflammation. When our barrier is compromised, we frequently experience irritation, redness, and pimples; however, applying a good moisturizer may help prevent this.

3. As We Age, The Skin Cell Cycle Lengthens.

As previously said, the usual skin cell cycle is 28 days, which means your skin sheds every month to reveal a new, healthy layer of skin. However, while our skin produces collagen naturally, it slows down over time, lengthening the cycle.

It Is critical to include an exfoliator in your skincare routine to avoid dull, dry, and rough skin. It aids in the removal of dead skin cells and keeps your skin supple and silky. Don't ignore your body! Use the body scrub 1-2 times a week to keep your skin smooth and healthy, and then seal in the moisture with hand and body lotion or body oil.

4. Being Proactive Pays Off.

Prevention, like anything else in life, is preferable to cure. The sooner you commit to a skincare program, the sooner you'll experience results. Premature aging, sun spots, and scars may all be avoided by taking care of your skin today.

It will also save you money in the long run since you will have less need for dermatologists and therapies to treat the impacts of poor skin habits, such as excessive sun exposure.

5. Skincare Products That Are Suitable For Your Skin Type

Each skin type has different demands, which is why it's critical to create a skincare regimen that's tailored to your specific challenges. It's natural for a product that worked for a friend (or someone on Instagram) to not work for you.

If you have dry, dehydrated skin, you should look for ultra-hydrating treatments that help your skin retain moisture. If you have combination skin, use different creams for your T-zone and cheeks. If you have acne or sensitive skin, calming, soothing lotions are your best bet. If you have oily skin, you should use treatments that absorb excess oil and balance out the skin tone.

6. It Complements Your Lifestyle.

Exercise, a balanced diet, and a good skincare routine are the winning combination for the cleanest, healthiest skin you've ever had!

Exercising frequently increases circulation, reduces stress, and adds shine to the skin, whereas a diet rich in whole foods provides your skin with the nutrition it requires to thrive. Add natural skincare to your daily regimen, and you'll be on your way to having the best skin you've ever had.

There are numerous advantages to using a skincare program, and the best one for you is determined by your skin type. To achieve the most glowing results, remember to nourish your face and body and stick to a new habit for at least a month.

CHOOSING THE BEST SKINCARE PRODUCTS FOR YOU

Choosing the best skincare products with the optimal ingredients for your skin requires a specialized approach. This requires a bit more time and patience, but it's well worth it.

Fortunately for you, we spoke with dermatologists to make the procedure less frightening. With this knowledge in your back pocket, you may feel more secure as a customer and perhaps avoid reactive skin disasters while trying new products in the future.

Understand Your Skin Type

According to cosmetic dermatologist Michele Green, MD, the most important factor in determining which skincare products will work best for you is your skin type. There are no inherently dangerous goods, but occasionally people with different skin types use the wrong product for their type of skin.

People with acne-prone or sensitive skin should be especially cautious when it comes to the ingredients in their skincare products. Oily skin, on the other hand, can handle a wider range of things that might cause breakouts or irritation in other skin types. La Roche-Posay's Effaclar Mat Mattifying Moisturizer is an excellent alternative for acne-prone individuals looking for a moisturizer for oily skin.

Most doctors recommends the following components for various skin types:

➢ Look for products containing alpha hydroxy acids (glycolic acid or salicylic acid), benzoyl peroxide, and hyaluronic acid if you have oily skin. These chemicals are efficient in controlling excess sebum production, whereas hyaluronic acid creates hydration just in areas that require it. An affordable face cleanser for oily skin that combines salicylic and hyaluronic acids is CeraVe Renewing SA Cleanser.

➢ Look for products containing shea butter and lactic acid if you have dry skin. These chemicals give hydration and gentle exfoliation to keep dry skin looking radiant.

➢ Look for products containing aloe vera, oats, and shea butter if you have sensitive skin. They're amazing moisturizers and usually don't break anyone out. Lipikar Wash AP+ by La Roche-Posay is a good drugstore body wash with shea butter for folks with dry, sensitive skin who want extra moisture.

If you're not sure what skin type you have, a visit to the dermatologist is in order. Once you've determined your skin type, you may begin selecting products with greater precision.

Don't Believe the Hype

Packaging and popularity are frequently easy traps that should not be given too much weight or relevance when deciding what to put on our skin. If you're going to buy a product based on a recommendation from a friend or influencer, consider not only how great their skin looks today, but also what sort of skin they had previously. This will provide you with a more reliable idea of how well the product will function for you.

In recent years, cult favorites like the St. Ives Apricot Scrub and several Mario Badescu products have faced lawsuits from customers who experienced severe adverse reactions. There's no need to worry if you have these goods in your cosmetics cupboard at home; they're not toxic for everyone. The reaction that certain well-known skincare companies and products have received may serve as a reminder that just because

something is popular does not mean it is popular for the right reasons or that it is the best product for you.

Regardless of how many positive ratings or stars the product has online, reading the ingredients list is always the best way to proceed.

LOOK FOR THESE INGREDIENTS

Most Skin doctors, considers glycerin to be the foundation of moisturizing products.

Ceramides and hyaluronic acid are both key moisturizing substances present naturally in the skin. Skin doctors loves hyaluronic acid serums but also search for glycerin and ceramides in lotions and creams.

L-Ascorbic acid (Vitamin C): Vitamin C, especially the l-ascorbic acid form, is an antioxidant that protects against UV damage and promotes collagen production.

Tocopherol (Vitamin E): Vitamin E has comparable properties to vitamin C and works best when paired as a skincare power duo. Augustinus Bader's The Hand Treatment combines Vitamin E, glycerin, and shea butter for a luxurious hand lotion.

Retinol: Retinol is a crucial ingredient to look for in products for your evening regimen. It works by transforming skin cells and stimulating collagen production.

Niacinamide (Vitamin B3): This chemical helps to reduce oil while also hydrating and evening out skin tone.

AVOID THESE ELEMENTS

Fragrance/Perfume: Added fragrances can cause skin allergies and irritation, therefore avoid them at all costs if you have sensitive skin.

Sulfates are washing chemicals that are commonly found in body washes and shampoos. They reduce the natural oil of the hair and skin and may irritate.

Parabens: Parabens are commonly employed as a chemical preservative in products to inhibit bacterial development. They're known as estrogen mimickers, which I and other industry professionals call them, and they may be harmful over time by disrupting hormonal balance. It is warned that this can be problematic for young children and individuals who are at risk of developing breast cancer.

Formaldehyde And Formaldehyde Releasers: Because formaldehyde is a known carcinogen, it is rarely shown in ingredient lists. However, it is frequently substituted by curiously named compounds (quaternion-15, DMDM hydantoin, diazolidinyl urea, imidazolidinyl urea) that slowly release formaldehyde to act as preservatives. It is unknown whether or not these compounds are dangerous in this capacity, however, they should be avoided as possible allergens.

Understand That Natural Does Not Always Imply Superior.

Although seeing familiar terminology in the ingredients list might be reassuring, it does not necessarily indicate the safest option. For example, poison ivy is a natural oil, but it's not one you want to rub all over your skin. I see people with reactions to natural essential oils quite regularly, so it's one of those things where everyone is different and you have to do what's best for yourself.

Natural and organic labels on product labels are sometimes more of a marketing ploy than anything else. Because those terms are not regulated and have no industry norms, they might deliver empty

promises. Furthermore, a product may be labeled as natural about only one or two of the ingredients on the list.

Pay Attention To The Order Of The Components.

Once you've determined which significant elements you want to avoid or pursue, pay attention to where they appear on the ingredients list. Looking at the first five components is a good rule of thumb, as they often account for roughly 80% of the product's composition.

Ingredients will be mentioned in order of greatest to lowest concentration, so if one of the first five ingredients is unpleasant or potentially irritating, you should avoid that product.

Similarly, if you're seeking certain components in a product, but those ingredients are only included at the end, the product isn't worth your money. The advantages of the compounds toward the end of the list will not be felt with such a small percentage of the total product.

Don't Be Alarmed By The Lengthy Ingredient List.

When it comes to the food we eat, we're usually taught to search for a shorter, more recognizable ingredient list. While a shorter list may be simpler to understand, it may not always be sufficient in terms of what you want from your skincare products.

When looking for anti-aging advantages or investing in medical-grade skincare, the ingredients list will certainly get longer. It should not dissuade you. Instead, seek assistance—either from a dermatologist or from technology—to assess if the product is a suitable fit for you.

Utilize Your Resources

You don't need to be a walking dictionary to choose skincare products with the right components. Utilize internet technologies to make your life easier.

Always Do A Patch Test.

A patch test is a good idea in your product elimination procedure. It's also a great reason to go to Ultra or Sephora without spending any money.

A patch test can help determine whether certain goods or substances are likely to trigger allergic responses, irritate your skin, or clog your pores.

"I believe the take-home message is: if it's hurting your skin in any way, stop using it; it's not the right product for you."

Testing all of your components before committing to them may take some time at first, but it will save you a lot of money and worry in the long run.

CHAPTER 4

SKIN-HEALTHY ACTIVITIES

10 Habits to Develop for Beautiful, Healthy Skin.

Many individuals spend a lot of money on cosmetics and skin care products to have a decent complexion. What they don't realize is that healthy and appealing skin starts with a regular skincare regimen.

This was shown in research on the developing purpose of skincare. The study found that a person's regular skin care practice has a positive impact on the overall quality of their complexion, especially if it is backed by effective products.

Here are 10 daily skincare routines for healthy, radiant skin to help you on your quest for a beautiful and bright complexion:

1. DRINK A LOT OF WATER

Drinking lots of water is not only the most fundamental skin care practice, but it is also a key habit for maintaining overall physical fitness. Our bodies' cells are mostly comprised of water, and water plays an important role in maintaining physiological equilibrium. Scientists have long studied the association between water and a healthy complexion based only on these parameters.

Drinking water will not only quench your thirst but will also keep your skin properly moisturized. New research published in the Journal of Clinical, Cosmetic, and Investigative Dermatology validates the skin-hydrating benefits of drinking enough water.

In the clinical experiment, 49 healthy women were divided into two groups. The patients in one group were encouraged to drink at least 5.2 liters of water per day, whereas the patients in the other group consumed less than 3.2 liters per day. After examining and evaluating the subjects'

skin hydration for a month, the researchers discovered that drinking a large amount of water every day significantly increases the moisture content of the skin.

Well-hydrated skin is transparent, with scarcely visible pores, and almost no imperfections, and looks radiant. Drinking water instead of coffee, juice, or other sweetened beverages is advised. Aside from its skin advantages, water is calorie-free, and drinking more of it may help you avoid calorie-rich drinks, allowing you to maintain a healthy weight.

2. USE SUNSCREEN

Sunscreen is any chemical or product that shields your skin from the UV rays of the sun. While getting a tan might make you feel more energized and attractive, you should avoid going out without sunscreen.

UV (ultraviolet) light from the sun has a major influence on the condition of your skin. In reality, most of the symptoms associated with skin aging are more typically the result of persistent exposure to sunlight than of one's actual age.

UV radiation causes skin drooping, stretching, and wrinkles by destroying the skin's elastic and collagen tissue. It also causes freckles, discoloration of the skin, age spots, and even skin cancer. Consider what your skin must go through when you go out in the sun without sunscreen.

For many years, sunscreen has been widely recognized for effectively preventing premature signs of skin aging. However, a recent study found that using sunscreen regularly had therapeutic effects on photo-

aged skin (or sun-damaged skin). Researchers observed that people who used sunscreen every day for 18 months had significant improvement in their skin health.

But keep in mind that sunscreen only works if you use the appropriate one and apply it correctly. The American Academy of Dermatology

(AAD) advises using a sunscreen with an SPF of 30 or higher that is water-resistant and protects against both UVA and UVB radiation. To keep protected, apply a generous amount of sunscreen to all exposed skin 15 minutes before going out and reapply every two hours.

3. EAT WELL.

Because your skin condition is a reflection of what is going on within your body, you must properly fuel your body to have a lovely and glowing complexion. This reality has long been understood, as various nutrition experts have demonstrated the positive relationship between adequate eating and youthful skin.

Given this, you should include skin-friendly meals in your skincare routine. Fruits and vegetables high in vitamin C are examples of such foods. This vitamin is well-known for its potent antioxidant properties, which protect the skin from the damaging effects of free radicals. Vitamin C has also been linked to faster skin healing and improved skin texture.

Vitamins A, E, and K, as well as selenium, omega-3, zinc, and monounsaturated and polyunsaturated fats (good fats), are all beneficial to your skin. So, the next time you design a meal plan, incorporate healthy servings of foods rich in critical nutrients.

4. PURCHASE BEAUTY SUPPLEMENTS

Eating your way to great skin is important; nevertheless, you must admit that it is difficult to get all of the nutrients your skin needs from the food you consume alone. Because your skin is the largest organ in your body, it needs more vitamins and minerals to be healthy.

Your skin Is regularly exposed to a variety of environmental factors that contribute to premature skin aging. So, in addition to increasing your regular vegetable and fruit consumption, it may be beneficial to take vitamins that help the skin. Multivitamins, particularly those containing vitamin E and biotin, antioxidants such as resveratrol, and hydration agents such as hyaluronic acid and collagen are all popular skin supplements.

Many studies have shown that beauty supplements, both oral and topical, can help enhance the quality and condition of your skin. One study on the impact of an antioxidant supplement on women's skin brightness found good results. After receiving a continuous daily dose of an antioxidant-rich oral supplement, the females who participated in the study had fewer skin imperfections, enhanced skin firmness, and more luminous skin.

Almonds, chamomile, green tea, and other botanical sources can also be used to give skincare benefits. Natural oils have antibacterial, anti-inflammatory, and other properties that aid in the prevention and treatment of skin diseases.

5. BEFORE GOING TO BED

Cleaning is an essential part of any skin care regimen. People have been cleaning their skin to enhance its health and appearance since ancient times. While cleaning technologies have evolved, the core concept has not: your skin requires cleansing.

You may not realize it, but your makeup is a free radical carrier in the environment. Even if you don't use makeup, your skin picks up dust and filth during the day, which sits on top of your perspiration and sebum.

When you don't clean your skin before bed, you're practically "sleeping with" free radicals. Free radicals damage the healthy collagen in your skin, causing fine lines and wrinkles.

In addition to causing harm to your skin, cosmetics, and oils can clog your facial pores. When this occurs, your skin is more prone to acne breakouts, enlarged pores, and other skin issues.

Facial cleaning is essential for maintaining a healthy and clear complexion. So, the next time you're tempted to sleep with your makeup on, remember the dangers and go for your facial cleanser, micellar water, or a face-cleaning wipe.

6. HAVE ENOUGH SLEEP

Getting adequate sleep (at least 7 hours per night) and not only resting should be an important part of your skincare routine. Whether you've read the studies or not, the connection between proper sleep and skin condition is undeniable. If you just sleep a few hours each night, you will soon see and feel negative impacts on your complexion.

The findings of research on common sleep problems and dermatological concerns emphasized the significant association between getting adequate sleep and skin conditions even more. The same study discovered that those who have sleep problems are more prone to acquire skin ailments such as eczema, psoriasis, and skin aging.

Sleep is essential for a healthy complexion since only deep and prolonged sleep allows your cells to regenerate and damaged cells to be repaired. Interrupting this process causes your skin to repair slowly, resulting in visible indications of aging. Allow your skin to age gracefully by getting your beauty rest.

7. CONTROL YOUR STRESS

Psychological stress is a major cause of many illnesses and has a big influence on your skin health. When you are nervous, your body produces "emergency" physiological reactions to help you deal with the

situation. Unfortunately, continuous stimulation of these processes has been linked to skin aging, among other things.

Skin aging is closely related to psychological stress. Stress causes immune system failure, DNA damage, and changes in endocrine and immunological control, all of which contribute to skin aging.

When you're continually anxious, your skin becomes more prone to microbial infection, in addition to aging. According to one clinical study, stress disrupts the antibacterial activity of the epidermis or the skin's outer layer. Infection becomes more likely if the skin's defensive mechanism is compromised.

Prevent all of these bad consequences by including stress management in your skin care regimen. To ease stress, try breathing exercises, listening to music, or aromatherapy. Topical applications of essential oils such as sweet almonds and chamomile might also be beneficial in this regard.

8. APPLY A MOISTURIZER

Some people believe that using a moisturizer is just for cosmetic purposes, while in fact, it is an essential aspect of skin maintenance.

Your skin is the most exposed area of your body, and this can cause dryness and moisture loss.

Applying moisturizer after cleaning, toning, or exfoliating is necessary to replace the skin's lost moisture and natural oils. Moisturized skin is silky, smooth, brighter, and more youthful-looking. Dehydrated skin, on the other hand, is dry, dull, and scaly – in other words, unappealing.

If you are afraid to incorporate moisturizing in your daily skincare routine because you have oily skin or live in a humid climate, experts advise you to do so. Instead of using cream-based moisturizers, try a lighter lotion or serum containing humectants like hyaluronic acid. Use a moisturizer that contains sunscreen for extra protection.

9. MAINTAIN YOUR BODY MOVEMENT

While exercise is typically connected with weight loss, an increasing number of individuals are finding how it improves healthy and youthful-looking skin. If you doubt this, look at athletes or those who lead an active lifestyle; don't they seem younger and have great skin?

Exercise helps to improve blood circulation. Walking, jogging, or dancing increases blood flow in the body. When this occurs, the nutrients in the blood are better transferred to your skin cells, resulting in well-nourished skin. Furthermore, improved blood flow assists in detoxification, resulting in a healthier complexion.

If you have skin inflammatory illnesses such as eczema or psoriasis, you should exercise with caution since an increase in body temperature might aggravate your condition. To minimize discomfort, exercise in a cool area, such as an air-conditioned gym, or jog at night rather than during the day. Swimming should also be avoided since the chlorine in the water might increase some of your symptoms.

10 . USE SKIN PRODUCTS WITH NATURAL INGREDIENTS.

Without skin care products, your regular skin care program would be incomplete. Contrary to popular belief, everyone needs and utilizes such items, whether they are aware of it or not. When using skin care products, be sure that the majority of the components are natural.

Botanical skin care products are safe, have anti-aging, anti-inflammatory, and antibacterial properties, and are even environmentally friendly. Cosmetics containing mostly man-made substances such as parabens, sulfates, phthalates, and formaldehyde, on the other hand, can cause skin diseases and damage.

Make it a habit to check the label to verify that you are only using skin care products derived from nature. Avoid the product at all costs if hazardous chemicals are found in the ingredients list.

CHAPTER 5
ACNE TREATMENT

WHAT EXACTLY IS ACNE?

Acne is a common skin ailment that results in pimples. You will almost always have pimples on your face. Acne is caused by clogged pores. Acne is most commonly associated with teenagers and young adults, however, it may occur in adults as well. There are treatments available to help you get rid of acne and avoid scarring. Acne vulgaris is the medical term for cane.

What Are the Different Types of Acne?

Acne comes in a variety of forms, including:

Pityrosporum folliculitis (fungal acne): Pityrosporum folliculitis occurs when yeast accumulates in your hair follicles. These may be uncomfortable and irritating.

Cystic Acne: Is characterized by deep, pus-filled pimples and nodules. Scarring can result from them.

Hormonal Acne: Adults with hormonal acne have an overproduction of sebum, which clogs their pores.

Nodular Acne: is a severe type of acne that causes pimples on the surface of your skin as well as sensitive, nodular lumps beneath your skin.

All of these types of acne can be damaging to your self-esteem, and both cystic and nodular acne can cause long-term skin damage in the form of scarring. It is recommended to get guidance from a healthcare specialist as soon as possible so that they can determine the best treatment option(s) for you.

Who Is Affected by Acne?

Acne affects almost everyone at some time in their lives. Acne is most common in teens and young adults who are going through hormonal changes, but it may also develop in adults. Adult acne is more prevalent in women and individuals who were designated female at birth (AFAB). If you have a family history of acne, you may be more likely to develop it.

What Is the Frequency of Acne?

If you have acne, realize that you are not alone. Acne is the most common skin condition that people face. An estimated 80% of people aged 11 to 30 have at least moderate acne.

Where Will My Acne Appear on My Body?

The most common places for acne to appear are on your:

• Face

• Front of the head

• Chest

• Shoulder blades

• The upper back

Oil glands may be found throughout your body. Acne is most frequent in locations with the most oil glands.

CAUSES AND SYMPTOMS

What Are The Acne Symptoms?

Acne symptoms on your skin include:

Pimples (pustules): Pimples packed with pus (papules).

Papules are small, discolored lumps that are typically red, purple, or deeper in color than your normal skin tone.

Blackheads are blocked pores with a dark top.

Whiteheads are blocked pores with a white surface.

Nodules are uncomfortable large bumps under your skin.

Cysts are painful fluid-filled (pus) masses beneath the skin.

Acne can be minor, resulting in a few occasional pimples, or severe, resulting in inflammatory papules. Nodules and cysts form as a result of severe acne.

What Are the Causes of Acne?

Acne is caused by clogged hair follicles or pores. Hair follicles are little tubes that hold a strand of hair. There are several glands in your body that drain into your hair follicles. A blockage develops when there is too much material inside your hair follicle. Your pores can get clogged with:

Sebum: An oily substance that acts as a barrier for your skin.

Bacteria: Bacteria normally present in small concentrations on your skin. If you have too many bacteria, your pores may become clogged.

Dead skin cells: Your skin cells shed often to make room for new cells to form. When your skin sheds dead skin cells, they can become entangled in your hair follicles.

When your pores clog, particles accumulate in your hair follicle, resulting in a pimple. This causes inflammation, which manifests as pain and swelling. Inflammation can also be seen as skin pigmentation, such as redness surrounding a pimple.

Acne Triggers

Certain elements in your environment, such as tight-fitting clothes and headgear, such as hats and sports helmets, might contribute to acne or aggravate an acne breakout.

• Air pollution and specific weather conditions, particularly high humidity.

• Using oily or greasy personal care products, such as heavy lotions and creams, or working in an environment where you frequently come into touch with grease, such as frying oil in a restaurant.

• Stress, which causes the hormone cortisol to rise.

• A medication side effect.

• Picking at your pimples.

Foods That Contribute to Acne

Some studies link specific foods and diets to acne, such as

• Skim milk.

• Protein derived from whey.

• High-sugar diets.

While high-sugar diets can cause acne, chocolate is not directly linked to acne.

To reduce your risk of acne, eat a balanced, healthy diet rich in fresh fruits and vegetables, particularly those high in vitamin C and beta-carotene, both of which help reduce inflammation.

Acne and Hormones

Acne is mostly a hormonal condition brought on by androgen hormones (testosterone). This usually becomes active during adolescence and

early adulthood. Acne may also emerge around the time of your menstruation as a result of hormonal activity. Acne can be caused by sensitivity to this hormone, as well as surface germs on your skin and substances generated by your body's glands.

DIAGNOSTIC AND TESTING

How Is Acne Diagnosis Made?

A skin exam can be used by a doctor to diagnose acne. During this examination, the physician will carefully examine your skin to learn more about your symptoms. Furthermore, they may inquire about acne risk factors such as:

• Are you stressed?

• Do you have an acne-prone family history?

• Do you have breakouts during your menstrual cycle as a woman or person AFAB?

• What drugs are you currently taking?

Your healthcare practitioner will not need to perform any diagnostic testing FOR mild acne, but if you have sudden, severe acne breakouts, especially if you're an adult, they may recommend tests to discover any underlying concerns.

Who Handles Acne?

Acne can be diagnosed and treated by a medical practitioner or a dermatologist. A dermatologist can assist you if you have persistent acne that is not improving with therapy.

How Bad Can Acne Get?

Dermatologists rank acne by severity:

Grade 1 (mild): Mostly whiteheads and blackheads, with a few papules and pustules.

Grade 2 (moderate or pustular acne): Multiple papules and pustules, mainly on your face.

Grade 3 (moderately severe or nodulocystic acne): Numerous papules and pustules, associated with sometimes inflammatory nodules. Your back and chest may also be impacted.

Grade 4 (severe nodulocystic acne): Numerous huge, painful, and inflammatory pustules and nodules.

TREATMENT AND MANAGEMENT

How Is Acne Handled?

Acne may be treated using a variety of methods. Each treatment option is different depending on your age, the type of acne you have, and its severity. To treat your skin, your doctor may advise you to take oral tablets, use topical drugs, or use medicated treatments. The goal of acne therapy is to prevent new pimples from forming and to heal existing blemishes on your skin.

Topical Acne Treatments

Your doctor may advise you to use a topical acne treatment to treat your skin. You can apply these drugs to your skin like you would a lotion or moisturizer. These might include anything containing one or more of the following ingredients:

Benzoyl Peroxide: This is available as an over-the-counter product as a leave-on gel or wash (such as Clearasil, Stridex, and PanOxyl). It targets surface bacteria, which are known to worsen acne. Lower concentrations and wash formulations are gentler on the skin.

Salicylic Acid: Is offered as an over-the-counter acne cleanser or lotion. It aids in the removal of the top layer of damaged skin. Salicylic acid eliminates dead skin cells, keeping your hair follicles clear.

Azelaic Acid: Is a natural acid present in many grains, including barley, wheat, and rye. It kills microorganisms on the skin and reduces edema.

Retinoids (vitamin A derivatives): Retinol, which is accessible without a prescription and includes Retin-A, Tazorac, and Differin, breaks up blackheads and whiteheads and helps prevent blocked pores, which are the earliest indicators of acne. The majority of persons are candidates for retinoid treatment. These drugs are not spot treatments and must be used on the entire afflicted region of the skin to prevent the formation of new pimples. You may need to use them for several months before seeing any beneficial outcomes.

Antibiotics: Topical medicines such as clindamycin and erythromycin decrease surface microorganisms that aggravate and cause acne. Antibiotics work better when combined with benzoyl peroxide.

Dapsone (Aczone): Is a topical gel that also has antibacterial properties. It provides relief from inflammatory acne.

Acne Medications Taken Orally

Oral acne medications are tablets that you take orally to treat your acne. Oral acne medications might include:

Antibiotics: Antibiotics are used to treat acne that is caused by bacteria. Tetracycline, minocycline, and doxycycline are common acne antibiotics. These are good for acne ranging from mild to severe.

Isotretinoin (Amnesteem, Claravis, and Sotret): An oral retinoid. Isotretinoin reduces the size of oil glands, which causes acne.

Contraceptives: Some contraceptives can occasionally help women and persons AFAB who suffer from acne. The Food and Drug Administration (FDA) of the United States has authorized a variety of birth control pills for the treatment of acne. Estrostep, Beyaz, Ortho Tri-Cyclen, and Yaz are some brand names. These tablets include a mix of estrogen (the primary AFAB sex hormone) and progesterone (a natural steroid that aids in menstrual regulation).

Hormone therapy: Hormone therapy can help some people with acne, especially if you have acne flare-ups or irregular periods caused by an excess of androgen (a hormone). Hormone treatment includes low-dose estrogen and progesterone (birth control pills) or spironolactone, a medication that reduces the influence of certain hormones on your hair follicles and oil glands.

Additional Acne Treatments

If topical or oral medications do not adequately treat your acne, or if you have acne scars, your healthcare practitioner may recommend one of many methods of acne therapy to clear your skin, including:

Steroids: Steroids can be used to treat severe acne by injecting them into large nodules to reduce inflammation.

Lasers: Lasers and light therapy are used to cure acne scars. A laser beam delivers heat to the scarred collagen beneath your skin. This is dependent on your body's wound-healing response to produce new, healthy collagen, which promotes the growth of new skin to replace it.

Chemical peels: This therapy removes the top layer of old skin by using particular chemicals. After removing the top layer of skin, new skin appears smoother and can help to reduce acne scars.

Antibiotics: How Do They Treat Acne?

Antibiotics are antibacterial medications. Some acne treatments might also reduce inflammation. Bacteria can block your pores, causing acne. Antibiotics are to blame for:

• Keeping microbes out of your body.

• Eliminating microorganisms.

• Preventing the growth of microorganisms.

If you have acne caused by bacteria or an infection, your doctor will prescribe antibiotics. Antibiotics treat infections caused by germs that enter a popped pimple, which can expand and become painful. This medication is not a cure for acne and should not be used long-term to treat acne.

How Can I Treat My Acne At Home?

• Washing your skin at least once daily with warm (not hot) water and a mild cleanser to help your acne go away. Cleansers are over-the-counter skin care products that aid in the cleaning of your skin.

• Washing your skin after exercising or sweating.

• Avoid using skin care products that contain alcohol, astringents, toners, or exfoliants, since they may irritate your skin.

• Take off your makeup at the end of the day or before bed.

• After cleaning, apply an oil-free moisturizer on your skin.

• Do not pop, pick, or squeeze your acne. Allow your skin to heal properly to avoid the formation of scars.

Consult a healthcare expert if your at-home skin care regimen isn't working to treat acne.

Is Acne Treatment Safe For Individuals Who Are Pregnant?

Many topical and oral acne solutions aren't safe to take during pregnancy. If you are pregnant or want to become pregnant, it is critical to discuss acne treatments with your doctor and tell them if you get pregnant.

How Long Does Acne Take To Clear Up?

Acne blemishes, on average, take one to two weeks to clear up on their own. You can speed up your body's healing process and help acne go gone faster with medicated treatment and a proper skin care routine. Even with medicine, it might take several weeks for severe acne to clear up.

PREVENTION

How Can I Avoid Acne?

Acne cannot be completely avoided, especially during hormonal changes, but you may reduce your chances of getting acne by:

• Washing your face daily with warm water and a facial cleanser.

• Applying a non-oily moisturizer.

• Using "noncomedogenic" cosmetics and removing them at the end of the day.

• Avoid touching your face with your hands.

PROGNOSIS / OUTLOOK

What Should I Do If I Have Acne?

Acne usually clears up by early adulthood, while some people struggle with acne throughout their lives. This condition can be managed with the assistance of your healthcare practitioner or a board-certified dermatologist. Various medications and treatments are viable therapeutic options. They target the underlying conditions that cause acne. It may take numerous treatments before you and your healthcare provider find one that works best for your skin. The skin care products that work for you may not work for someone else who has similar problems.

Can Acne Cause Scars?

Yes, acne may occasionally leave scars. This occurs when acne penetrates your skin's top layer and affects deeper skin layers. Inflammation causes your acne pores to enlarge and the pore walls to collapse, causing skin damage. Scarring might be frightening, which is understandable. Your doctor will determine the type of acne that created your scars before treating you. There are several acne scar treatment treatments available.

What Impact Does Acne Have on My Mental Health?

Acne can disturb your mental health since it impacts your appearance and self-esteem. Acne growth is frequently out of your control if hormones cause it. This might cause stress, which can affect subsequent breakouts. Teenagers and young adults can struggle with acne. Consult a healthcare professional or a mental health specialist if your acne makes you worried or prevents you from engaging in social activities with your friends and family.

When Should I Visit My Physician?

Consult a doctor as soon as you notice pimples so that you may begin treatment before scarring develops. Consult a doctor if you're using an acne treatment that isn't clearing up your acne or causing skin irritation, such as itching or skin discoloration.

What Should I Inquire of My Doctor?

• Which type of acne do I have?

• How bad is my acne?

• Should I see a dermatologist?

• What OTC medications do you recommend?

• Which prescription medications do you recommend?

Acne is the most common skin condition, and it can have an impact on your mental health and self-esteem. Consult a healthcare specialist or a dermatologist if you have persistent acne. If at-home skin care methods do not work, your acne may require a little more help to clear up with medication. While it may be tempting, avoid picking at your acne or popping pimples to avoid scarring. Remember that acne is temporary and will go away with the right treatment tailored to your skin.

SUMMARY

All of the basic skin care tips listed above may appear too simple to be effective, but they are supported by science. If you believe you are willing to undergo painful dermatological procedures just to have younger-looking skin, why not try these simple things that can help you achieve the same results?

Even Hollywood celebrities have stated that the aforementioned skincare routine works. However, keep in mind that the skin-improving benefits will only be achieved if you include these activities in your regular beauty regimen. Finally, when it comes to skincare, consistency is everything!

www.ingramcontent.com/pod-product-compliance
Lightning Source LLC
Chambersburg PA
CBHW071006260726
48661CB00007B/2823